NOOM DIET RECIPES

Key Principles Of The Noom Diet Nourishment For Body And Mind And 100 Healthy, Delicious, Flexible Recipes For Every Day

CONTENTS

INTRODUCTION

Welcome to "NOOM Diet Recipes," a culinary journey that combines the principles of the NOOM diet with a diverse array of delicious, healthy, and flexible recipes. In this book, we embark on a culinary adventure that not only nourishes the body but also tantalizes the taste buds.

A. Brief Overview of the NOOM Diet Approach:

The NOOM diet is not just another fad diet; it's a comprehensive approach to healthy living that focuses on sustainable weight loss and overall well-being. Unlike restrictive diets that eliminate entire food groups or require meticulous calorie counting, NOOM emphasizes a balanced approach to eating. It encourages mindful eating, portion control, and making healthier food choices without depriving oneself of the foods they love. NOOM promotes a positive relationship with food, aiming for long-term success rather than short-term fixes.

B. Importance of Incorporating Healthy, Delicious, and Flexible Recipes into Daily Routine:

Eating healthily doesn't have to mean sacrificing flavor or satisfaction. By incorporating delicious and nutritious recipes into your daily routine, you can achieve your health goals without feeling deprived. The key is to find recipes that not only align with the principles of the NOOM diet but also excite your taste buds and fit seamlessly into your lifestyle. With the right recipes, healthy eating becomes enjoyable and sustainable, making it easier to stick to your health and wellness goals in the long run.

C. Purpose of the Book: To Provide a Diverse Collection of 100 Recipes Suitable for the NOOM Diet:

The purpose of "NOOM Diet Recipes" is simple: to provide you with a treasure trove of culinary delights that support your NOOM journey. Whether you're craving hearty breakfasts, satisfying lunches, flavorful dinners, or indulgent desserts, this book has you covered. With a collection of 100 recipes carefully curated to align with the principles of the NOOM diet, you'll never run out of delicious and healthy meal ideas. From vibrant salads to comforting soups, from savory stir-fries to decadent treats, each recipe is designed to nourish both body and soul while keeping you on track with your health goals.

So, let's embark on this culinary adventure together and discover how delicious and satisfying healthy eating can truly be with "NOOM Diet Recipes."

BREAKFAST RECIPES

A. Introduction to Breakfast on the NOOM Diet:

Breakfast is often hailed as the most important meal of the day, and rightly so, especially when following the NOOM Diet. As you embark on your NOOM journey, it's crucial to kickstart your day with a nutritious breakfast that sets the tone for healthy choices throughout the day. The breakfast recipes in this chapter are carefully curated to not only tantalize your taste buds but also align with the principles of the NOOM Diet, promoting sustainable weight loss and overall well-being.

B. Delicious and Healthy Breakfast Options:

1. Beginner-Friendly Smoothie Recipes

Smoothies are a fantastic way to pack a plethora of nutrients into one convenient and delicious drink. Whether you're rushing out the door or leisurely enjoying your morning routine, these beginner-friendly smoothie recipes will keep you energized and satisfied throughout the morning. From classic green blends to vibrant berry concoctions, there's a smoothie to suit every taste preference and dietary requirement.

2. Colorful Fruit Bowls with Nutritious Toppings

Fuel your body with a burst of color and flavor by indulging in vibrant fruit bowls topped with nutritious accouterments. These bowls not only provide a visually stunning start to your day but also offer a plethora of vitamins, minerals, and antioxidants. Whether adorned with crunchy granola, creamy Greek yogurt, or a drizzle of honey, these fruit bowls are as versatile as they are delicious, making them a perfect addition to your breakfast repertoire.

3. Quick and Easy Overnight Oats Variations

Simplify your mornings with the convenience of overnight oats, a no-fuss breakfast option that can be prepared in advance and customized to suit your taste preferences. From decadent chocolate peanut butter to refreshing tropical mango coconut, these overnight oats variations are sure to tantalize your taste buds while keeping you full and satisfied until lunchtime. Prepare them the night before, pop them in the fridge, and wake up to a nutritious and delicious breakfast that's ready to enjoy.

C. Benefits of Starting the Day with a Balanced Breakfast:

Starting your day with a balanced breakfast sets the stage for making healthier choices throughout the day. By fueling your body with a nutritious morning meal, you provide it with the energy and nutrients it needs to function optimally. Additionally, eating breakfast can help regulate appetite, prevent overeating later in the day, and improve overall mood and cognition. Incorporating these delicious and healthy breakfast options into your routine not only supports your weight loss goals but also promotes a happier and healthier lifestyle. So, embrace the power of breakfast on the NOOM Diet and kickstart your day the right way.

SAVORING NOON WITH NUTRITIOUS LUNCH RECIPES

A fulfilling and wholesome lunch is not just a meal; it's a vital part of our daily routine. It provides the necessary fuel to power through the rest of the day, ensuring sustained energy levels and mental alertness. In the realm of the NOOM Diet, lunch holds a special significance as it sets the tone for the remainder of the day's eating habits. Let's delve into why a satisfying and nutritious lunch is paramount, explore simple yet delectable lunch ideas, and uncover the art of meal prepping for busy weekdays.

Importance of a Satisfying and Nutritious Lunch:

Lunch is the midday recharge we all need. It's not merely about satisfying hunger pangs but also about replenishing vital nutrients to support overall well-being. A balanced lunch can stabilize blood sugar levels, enhance cognitive function, and even contribute to weight management by preventing overeating later in the day. Moreover, a satisfying lunch can boost productivity and mood, making it an essential aspect of self-care in our hectic lives.

Simple and Tasty Lunch Ideas:

1. Colorful Salads with Protein-Rich Toppings:

Salads are a quintessential lunch option, offering a plethora of nutrients and flavors in one bowl. Start with a base of leafy greens such as spinach or kale, then add a variety of colorful vegetables like bell peppers, tomatoes, and cucumbers. To elevate the protein content, incorporate lean sources such as grilled chicken breast, tofu, or chickpeas. Finish with a sprinkle of nuts or seeds for added crunch and a drizzle of homemade vinaigrette for a burst of flavor.

2. Flavorful Wraps or Sandwiches with Fresh Ingredients:

Wraps and sandwiches are versatile lunchtime favorites that can be customized to suit individual preferences. Opt for whole-grain wraps or bread as a nutritious base. Fill them with an assortment of fresh ingredients such as sliced turkey or roast beef, avocado, lettuce, and hummus. Experiment with different spreads and condiments to enhance taste without compromising on health. These handheld delights are convenient for on-the-go lunches without sacrificing nutritional value.

3. Hearty Soups and Stews for a Filling Midday Meal:

Nothing beats the comfort of a warm bowl of soup or stew during lunchtime. Packed with vegetables, lean proteins, and flavorful broths, soups and stews offer a satisfying and nourishing option. Prepare a batch over the weekend and portion it into individual servings for quick reheating throughout the week. Experiment with diverse ingredients and spices to create tantalizing variations that cater to your taste buds while adhering to NOOM Diet principles.

Tips for Meal Prepping Lunches for Busy Weekdays:

Efficient meal prepping is the key to ensuring that nutritious lunches are readily available, even on the busiest of weekdays. Here are some tips to streamline the process:

Plan your meals ahead: Take some time each week to plan your lunch menu. Consider incorporating a variety of recipes to keep things interesting while meeting your nutritional goals.

Batch cooking: Prepare larger quantities of lunch items, such as salads, soups, or protein sources, and portion them into individual containers for easy grab-and-go meals throughout the week.

Invest in quality storage containers: Invest in durable, airtight containers to store prepped ingredients and meals safely. Opt for BPA-free options that are microwave and dishwasher safe for added convenience.

Utilize versatile ingredients: Choose ingredients that can be used in multiple recipes to minimize waste and simplify meal prep. For example, roast a batch of vegetables that can be added to salads, wraps, or served as a side dish.

Schedule meal prep time: Designate a specific day or time each week dedicated to meal prepping. Treat it as a non-negotiable appointment to ensure consistency and success.

By embracing the importance of a satisfying and nutritious lunch and incorporating simple yet flavorful recipes into your repertoire, you can nourish your body and mind while adhering to the principles of the NOOM Diet. With strategic meal prepping, even the busiest of weekdays can be navigated effortlessly, ensuring that wholesome lunches are always within reach. So, let's embark on this culinary journey together and elevate our lunchtime experience to new heights of health and satisfaction.

NOURISHING DINNERS FOR HEALTH AND FLAVOR

As the sun sets and the day draws to a close, there's a unique opportunity to indulge in a meal that not only satisfies our hunger but also nourishes our bodies. Dinner holds a special place in our daily routines, offering a moment to unwind and refuel after a busy day. In this chapter, we delve into the realm of dinner recipes tailored to support your Noom journey—recipes that not only tantalize the taste buds but also promote overall health and wellness.

A. Significance of a Balanced Dinner for Overall Health:

The importance of a balanced dinner cannot be overstated. It serves as the foundation for replenishing nutrients, regulating metabolism, and supporting bodily functions as we prepare for rest. A well-balanced dinner should encompass lean proteins, vibrant vegetables, whole grains, and healthy fats, providing a harmonious blend of macronutrients and micronutrients essential for optimal health.

B. Mouthwatering Dinner Options Suitable for Beginners:

Embarking on a culinary journey can be daunting, especially for beginners. Fear not, for the realm of dinner recipes offers a plethora of delightful options that are both approachable and satisfying. Let's explore some delectable choices:

1. Lean Protein-Based Dishes with Colorful Vegetable Sides

Grilled lemon herb chicken with roasted sweet potatoes and steamed broccoli

Baked salmon with quinoa pilaf and sautéed spinach

Turkey meatballs served with zucchini noodles and marinara sauce

2. One-Pot Meals for Easy Cleanup and Preparation

Hearty vegetable and lentil stew   - Chicken and vegetable stir-fry with brown rice

Shrimp and quinoa skillet with bell peppers and onions

3. Creative Ways to Incorporate Whole Grains into Dinner Recipes

Veggie-loaded whole wheat pasta primavera

Quinoa and black bean stuffed bell peppers

Mediterranean-inspired bulgur salad with chickpeas and fresh herbs

C. Importance of Portion Control and Mindful Eating During Dinner

Amidst the aroma of savory dishes and the temptation to indulge, it's crucial to practice mindful eating and portion control during dinner. Paying attention to hunger cues, savoring each bite, and being mindful of portion sizes can help prevent overeating and promote a healthier relationship with food. Remember, it's not just about what you eat but how you eat it.

Incorporating these principles into your dinner routine can pave the way for a more balanced and fulfilling lifestyle. Let your dinner table be a sanctuary of nourishment, where every bite is savored and every meal is a celebration of health and flavor.

THE STOPLIGHT COLOR HACK

A. Introduction to the Stoplight Color System:

Welcome to the world of the Stoplight Color Hack—a revolutionary approach to making healthier food choices. Imagine having a simple, intuitive system that guides you towards nutritious options every time you prepare a meal or go grocery shopping. That's precisely what the Stoplight Color System offers.

Inspired by the familiar traffic light signals, this system categorizes foods into three color-coded groups: green, yellow, and red. Each color corresponds to the nutritional value and healthiness of the food, providing a straightforward way to assess and prioritize your dietary decisions.

Green signifies foods that are packed with essential nutrients, low in calories, and highly beneficial for your overall health. These include fruits, vegetables, whole grains, lean proteins, and healthy fats—the foundation of a balanced diet.

Yellow indicates foods that should be consumed in moderation. While they may offer some nutritional benefits, they may also contain higher levels of sugar, salt, or unhealthy fats. Examples include certain dairy products, processed meats, and refined carbohydrates.

Red flags foods that are high in calories, sugar, unhealthy fats, or sodium and offer minimal nutritional value. These are typically highly processed, sugary snacks, fried foods, sugary beverages, and other unhealthy indulgences that should be limited or avoided altogether.

B. Explanation of How It Aids in Making Healthier Food Choices:

The beauty of the Stoplight Color Hack lies in its simplicity. By visually categorizing foods into green, yellow, and red, it provides a clear framework for assessing their nutritional value at a glance. This makes it easier to prioritize nutrient-dense foods while being mindful of those that should be consumed sparingly.

Moreover, the Stoplight Color System empowers you to develop a deeper understanding of the nutritional content of various foods. Over time, you'll become more adept at making informed choices, leading to a healthier diet and lifestyle.

By incorporating more green foods into your meals and minimizing consumption of yellow and red foods, you'll naturally increase your intake of essential nutrients, fiber, and antioxidants while reducing your consumption of empty calories, unhealthy fats, and added sugars.

C. Practical Tips for Implementing the Stoplight Color Hack in Daily Meals:

Implementing the Stoplight Color Hack in your daily meals is easier than you might think. Here are some practical tips to help you get started:

1. Plan Your Meals: Before heading to the grocery store, take some time to plan your meals for the week. Aim to include a variety of green foods in each meal, supplemented by smaller portions of yellow foods and minimal amounts of red foods.

2. Shop Smart: When shopping for groceries, focus on filling your cart with predominantly green foods, such as fresh produce, whole grains, and lean proteins. Be selective when it comes to yellow and red foods, opting for healthier options whenever possible.

3. Plate It Right: When plating your meals, aim to fill at least half of your plate with green foods, such as vegetables and whole grains. Use the remaining space for smaller portions of yellow and red foods, keeping proportions in mind.

4. Snack Wisely: When snacking, reach for nutrient-dense options like fresh fruit, nuts, yogurt, or hummus with veggies. If you're craving something indulgent, opt for smaller portions of yellow or red snacks and savor them mindfully.

5. Stay Consistent: Consistency is key to seeing results with the Stoplight Color Hack. Aim to make healthier choices the norm rather than the exception, and don't be too hard on yourself if you occasionally indulge in yellow or red foods.

D. Testimonials or Success Stories Showcasing the Effectiveness of the Stoplight Color Hack:

Here are some testimonials from individuals who have successfully implemented the Stoplight Color Hack into their lives:

"I've struggled with maintaining a healthy diet for years, but the Stoplight Color System has been a game-changer for me. It's made me more conscious of what I eat, and I've noticed a significant improvement in my energy levels and overall well-being." - Sarah

"As a busy parent, I've always found it challenging to make nutritious meals for my family. But with the Stoplight Color Hack, meal planning has become so much simpler. My kids even enjoy helping me choose green foods at the grocery store!" - David

"After years of yo-yo dieting, I finally feel like I've found a sustainable approach to healthy eating with the Stoplight Color System. It's helped me break free from restrictive diets and develop a more balanced relationship with food." - Emily

These testimonials serve as inspiring examples of how the Stoplight Color Hack can empower individuals to make healthier food choices and transform their lives for the better. By incorporating this intuitive system into your daily routine, you too can embark on a journey towards improved health and vitality.

DESSERTS AND TREATS

In the world of dieting, desserts and treats often carry a stigma of guilt and indulgence. However, within the realm of the Noom Diet, we embrace a different approach—one that allows for enjoyment without compromise. In this chapter, we delve into Noom-friendly dessert options, explore recipes for mindful indulgence, and provide strategies for managing cravings and nurturing a sweet tooth in a healthy way.

A. Noom-friendly Dessert Options:

Gone are the days of deprivation and restriction. The Noom Diet encourages a balanced approach to eating, which includes satisfying your sweet tooth without sabotaging your goals. By incorporating nutrient-dense ingredients and mindful portion control, you can indulge in desserts guilt-free.

From creamy yogurt parfaits adorned with fresh fruit to decadent dark chocolate avocado mousse, there's a plethora of Noom-friendly dessert options to tantalize your taste buds. By focusing on whole foods and minimizing added sugars, these desserts not only satisfy cravings but also provide essential nutrients to support your overall well-being.

B. Mindful Indulgence Recipes:

Indulgence doesn't have to equate to overindulgence. With mindful eating practices, you can savor every bite of your favorite treats while staying attuned to your body's hunger and fullness cues.

Explore the art of mindful indulgence through recipes that prioritize quality ingredients and intentional enjoyment. From homemade granola bars bursting with nuts and dried fruits to baked apples drizzled with cinnamon and honey, these recipes are designed to nourish both body and soul.

By slowing down and savoring each mouthful, you can cultivate a deeper appreciation for the flavors and textures of your desserts, making every indulgence a truly gratifying experience.

C. Strategies for Managing Cravings and Sweet Tooth:

Cravings are a natural part of life, but they don't have to derail your progress on the Noom Diet. By understanding the root causes of cravings and adopting strategies to address them, you can navigate temptations with ease.

Learn how to differentiate between physical hunger and emotional cravings, and discover alternative ways to cope with stress or boredom that don't involve reaching for sugary treats. Incorporate mindfulness techniques such as deep breathing and meditation to cultivate greater awareness of your body's signals and respond to them in a healthful manner.

Additionally, experiment with flavor combinations and textures to satisfy your sweet tooth in a nutritious way. Whether it's blending frozen bananas into creamy "nice" cream or sprinkling unsweetened cocoa powder over Greek yogurt, there are endless possibilities for indulgence within the framework of the Noom Diet.

UNDERSTANDING THE NOOM DIET

In the world of health and wellness, the NOOM Diet has emerged as a refreshing approach that goes beyond mere restriction and calorie counting. It's not just about shedding pounds; it's about fostering a sustainable and healthy relationship with food. So, what exactly is the NOOM Diet, and why is it gaining so much attention?

A. Explanation of the NOOM Diet Principles:

At its core, the NOOM Diet revolves around the principle of behavior change. Unlike traditional diets that focus solely on what you eat, NOOM takes into account the why and how of eating. It emphasizes understanding the psychological triggers behind our food choices and developing healthier habits for the long term.

One of the key features of the NOOM Diet is its use of a color-coded system to classify foods. This system categorizes foods into green, yellow, and red categories based on their calorie density and nutritional value. Green foods are low in calories but high in nutrients, while yellow foods are moderately calorie-dense, and red foods are higher in calories and often low in nutritional value. By encouraging a higher consumption of green foods and moderation with yellow and red foods, the NOOM Diet promotes a balanced approach to eating.

B. Emphasis on Balanced Nutrition and Mindful Eating:

Another fundamental aspect of the NOOM Diet is its emphasis on balanced nutrition. Rather than demonizing certain food groups or macronutrients, NOOM encourages a well-rounded diet that includes a variety of foods from all food groups. This approach ensures that your body receives the essential nutrients it needs for optimal health and function.

Mindful eating is also a cornerstone of the NOOM Diet. This involves paying attention to the sensory experience of eating, such as the taste, texture, and aroma of food, as well as recognizing hunger and fullness cues. By practicing mindfulness during meals and snacks, individuals can develop a greater awareness of their eating habits and make more conscious choices.

C. Flexibility and Sustainability as Key Components:

One of the most appealing aspects of the NOOM Diet is its flexibility. Unlike rigid diet plans that dictate what and when you can eat, NOOM encourages individuals to make choices that align with their personal preferences, cultural backgrounds, and lifestyle. This flexibility allows for greater adherence to the diet and makes it easier to sustain in the long term.

Sustainability is another critical component of the NOOM Diet. Rather than promoting quick fixes or drastic weight loss measures, NOOM focuses on making gradual, sustainable changes that can be maintained over time. By setting realistic goals and implementing small changes consistently, individuals can achieve lasting results without feeling deprived or overwhelmed.

In summary, the NOOM Diet offers a fresh perspective on weight loss and healthy eating. By focusing on behavior change, balanced nutrition, mindful eating, flexibility, and sustainability, it provides a holistic approach to achieving and maintaining a healthy lifestyle. In the following chapters, we'll delve deeper into the practical aspects of the NOOM Diet, including delicious recipes and meal plans to support your journey towards better health and well-being.

PLANNING FOR SUCCESS

In the realm of achieving dietary goals, success is often found not in sporadic efforts but in consistent planning and preparation. In this chapter, we delve into the vital aspects of meal planning, grocery shopping, and mindful eating practices essential for adhering to the NOOM diet.

A. Tips for Meal Planning and Preparation:

1. Set Clear Goals: Before embarking on your meal planning journey, define your objectives. Whether it's weight loss, better nutrition, or simply adopting a healthier lifestyle, having clear goals will guide your meal choices and portion sizes.

2. Create a Weekly Menu: Planning your meals for the week ahead can save time, money, and unnecessary stress. Sit down and sketch out a menu for breakfast, lunch, dinner, and snacks, ensuring variety and balance in your choices.

3. Consider Nutritional Balance: Aim for a diverse range of foods that provide essential nutrients. Incorporate plenty of fruits, vegetables, lean proteins, whole grains, and healthy fats into your meals to meet your body's needs.

4. Batch Cooking: Allocate time each week for batch cooking. Prepare large quantities of staple foods like grains, beans, and proteins that can be easily incorporated into different dishes throughout the week, saving you time on busy days.

5. Portion Control: Invest in portion-controlled containers or use measuring cups to ensure you're not overeating. Learning to recognize appropriate portion sizes can help prevent overconsumption and aid in weight management.

B. Grocery Shopping Guide for NOOM-Friendly Ingredients:

1. Focus on Whole Foods: When navigating the grocery aisles, prioritize whole, nutrient-dense foods over processed options. Fresh fruits and vegetables, lean proteins, whole grains, and healthy fats should form the foundation of your shopping list.

2. Colorful Produce: Make it a point to fill your cart with a rainbow of fruits and

vegetables. Different colors indicate varying nutrient profiles, so aim for a diverse selection to maximize nutritional intake.

3. Lean Proteins: Opt for lean sources of protein such as poultry, fish, tofu, legumes, and low-fat dairy products. These options are not only rich in protein but also lower in saturated fats, making them ideal choices for a balanced diet.

4. Whole Grains: Choose whole grains like brown rice, quinoa, barley, and whole wheat bread over refined grains. Whole grains are higher in fiber and nutrients, providing sustained energy and promoting digestive health.

5. Healthy Fats: Incorporate sources of healthy fats such as avocados, nuts, seeds, and olive oil into your shopping list. These fats are essential for heart health and help keep you feeling full and satisfied.

C. Importance of Portion Control and Mindful Eating Practices:

1. Listen to Your Body: Practice mindful eating by paying attention to hunger and fullness cues. Eat slowly, savoring each bite, and stop when you feel satisfied, rather than stuffed.

2. Use Smaller Plates: Trick your brain into eating smaller portions by using smaller plates and bowls. This visual illusion can help

prevent overeating and promote better portion control.

3. Avoid Distractions: Minimize distractions while eating, such as watching TV or scrolling through your phone. Focus on the taste, texture, and aroma of your food, allowing yourself to fully enjoy the eating experience.

4. Stay Hydrated: Sometimes thirst can masquerade as hunger. Stay hydrated throughout the day by drinking plenty of water, herbal teas, or infused water to prevent unnecessary snacking.

5. Practice Moderation: Remember that no food is inherently good or bad. Allow yourself to indulge occasionally in your favorite treats,

but practice moderation and balance in your overall diet.

By incorporating these strategies into your routine, you'll be well-equipped to navigate the challenges of meal planning, grocery shopping, and portion control on your NOOM diet journey. With careful planning and mindful eating practices, success is within reach, paving the way for a healthier, happier you.

RECIPE SECTIONS

In the realm of culinary delight, the recipe sections of the "NOOM DIET RECIPES" cookbook beckon with promises of nourishment, flavor, and satisfaction. Each section is meticulously crafted to cater to various moments throughout the day, ensuring that every mealtime becomes an opportunity to embrace wholesome eating without sacrificing taste. Let's delve into the delectable offerings awaiting you within each category:

A. Breakfast Delights:

1. Nutritious and satisfying breakfast recipes to start the day right:

Rise and shine to a plethora of morning marvels designed to fuel your day with vitality. From vibrant smoothie bowls bursting with fruits and superfoods to hearty oatmeal brimming with wholesome grains and toppings, these breakfast creations are a testament to the art of starting the day on the right note.

2. Options for both quick weekday mornings and leisurely weekend brunches:

Whether you're racing against the clock on a bustling weekday morning or relishing the unhurried pace of a weekend brunch, our recipes cater to every tempo. Dive into swift and savory egg muffins or linger over fluffy pancakes adorned with fresh berries – the choice is yours, no matter the hour.

B. Lunchtime Favorites:

1. Flavorful and filling lunch recipes suitable for work or home:

Midday meals become moments of culinary bliss with our array of lunchtime favorites. From vibrant salads brimming with crisp vegetables and protein-packed grains to hearty soups that warm the soul, these recipes are crafted to satisfy hunger and tantalize taste buds, whether enjoyed at the office desk or in the comfort of home.

2. Portable options for on-the-go convenience:

Embrace the hustle and bustle of life with our selection of portable lunchtime delights. From wholesome wraps filled with colorful veggies and lean proteins to satisfying grain bowls bursting with flavor, these recipes ensure that nourishment accompanies you wherever your day takes you.

C. Dinner Creations:

1. Wholesome and delicious dinner recipes for weeknight meals:

End your day on a high note with our collection of dinner creations designed to simplify mealtime without compromising on taste. From quick and easy stir-fries to comforting one-pot wonders, these recipes transform weeknight dinners into moments of culinary triumph.

2. Variety of cuisines and flavors to keep dinner time exciting:

Explore the rich tapestry of global flavors with our diverse range of dinner recipes. Whether you're craving the spicy warmth of a Mexican-inspired dish or the fragrant aromas of an Asian-inspired stir-fry, our recipes invite you to embark on a culinary journey from the comfort of your own kitchen.

D. Snacks and Sides:

1. Nourishing snack options to curb cravings between meals:

Banish midday munchies with our selection of nourishing snack options. From crunchy veggie sticks paired with creamy hummus to homemade trail mix bursting with nuts and dried fruits, these snacks offer a satisfying solution to cravings without derailing your dietary goals.

2. Healthy side dishes to complement any main course:

Elevate your meals with our array of healthy side dishes designed to complement any main course. From vibrant roasted vegetables seasoned to perfection to wholesome grain salads bursting with flavor, these recipes add an extra layer of nutrition and taste to every plate.

E. Sweet Treats:

1. Indulgent yet guilt-free dessert recipes for satisfying cravings:

Satisfy your sweet tooth without the guilt with our selection of indulgent yet wholesome dessert recipes. From decadent chocolate avocado mousse to refreshing fruit sorbets, these sweet treats offer a guilt-free way to indulge in a moment of culinary decadence.

2. Lower-calorie alternatives to traditional sweets:

Rediscover the joy of dessert with our collection of lower-calorie alternatives to traditional sweets. From light and airy angel food cake to refreshing fruit skewers drizzled with honey, these recipes prove that you can have your cake and eat it too, all while staying true to your dietary goals.

In the pages that follow, prepare to embark on a culinary journey filled with flavor, nourishment, and endless possibilities. With the "NOOM DIET RECIPES" cookbook as your guide, every meal becomes an opportunity to savor the joys of wholesome eating, one delicious bite at a time.

RECIPE FEATURES

Welcome to the heart of the Noom Diet Recipes book! In this chapter, we'll delve into the essential features that make each recipe not only delicious but also tailored to support your health and dietary goals. From nutritional information to cooking tips and serving suggestions, we've got you covered on every aspect to ensure your culinary journey is both satisfying and beneficial.

A. Nutritional Information for Each Recipe:

Understanding the nutritional value of the food you consume is crucial for maintaining a balanced diet. That's why each recipe in this book comes with detailed nutritional information. From calories and macronutrients to vitamins and minerals, you'll have a comprehensive breakdown of what you're eating, empowering you to make informed choices that align with your health objectives.

B. Dietary Modifications and Substitutions:

We recognize that everyone's dietary needs and preferences are unique. Whether you're following a specific eating plan, managing food allergies, or simply want to explore alternative ingredients, we've included modifications and substitutions for every recipe. Whether you're vegan, gluten-free, or looking to reduce sodium intake, you'll find adaptable options that cater to your specific requirements without compromising on flavor or satisfaction.

C. Cooking Tips and Techniques:

Cooking is both an art and a science, and mastering the right techniques can elevate your dishes to new heights. In this chapter, you'll discover a wealth of cooking tips and techniques designed to enhance flavor and texture while maintaining the nutritional integrity of each recipe. From proper seasoning and marinating to cooking methods that maximize taste and minimize added fats, you'll learn valuable skills that will make every meal a culinary delight.

D. Serving Suggestions and Pairing Ideas:

No meal is complete without thoughtful presentation and complementary flavors. That's why we've included serving suggestions and pairing ideas for each recipe, helping you create well-balanced and satisfying meals. Whether you're planning a cozy dinner for two or hosting a gathering with friends and family, you'll find inspiration for creating harmonious combinations that tantalize the taste buds and nourish the body.

In summary, the recipe features outlined in this chapter are designed to empower you on your journey towards a healthier and more fulfilling lifestyle. With nutritional information, dietary modifications, cooking tips, and serving suggestions at your fingertips, you'll be equipped to create delicious meals that support your wellness goals while satisfying your cravings. So, roll up your sleeves, gather your ingredients, and let's embark on a culinary adventure that celebrates the joy of nourishing both body and soul with Noom Diet Recipes.

TIPS FOR SUSTAINABLE WEIGHT LOSS

In the pursuit of weight loss, sustainability is key. Crash diets and extreme measures may offer rapid results, but they often lead to rebound weight gain and can be detrimental to your overall health. In this chapter, we'll explore essential tips for achieving sustainable weight loss through the lens of incorporating physical activity, overcoming challenges and setbacks, and prioritizing self-care and mental well-being.

A. Incorporating Physical Activity into Daily Routines:

Exercise isn't just about burning calories; it's about improving overall health and well-being. Incorporating physical activity into your daily routine is crucial for sustainable weight loss. Here are some tips to help you get moving:

1. Find activities you enjoy: Whether it's dancing, hiking, swimming, or yoga, choose activities that you genuinely enjoy. This makes it easier to stick to your exercise routine long-term.

2. Start small and gradually increase intensity: Don't feel pressured to jump into high-intensity workouts right away. Start with manageable activities and gradually increase the intensity as your fitness level improves.

3. Make it a habit: Schedule regular exercise sessions just like any other appointment. Consistency is key to seeing results.

4. Stay active throughout the day: Look for opportunities to sneak in extra activity throughout the day, such as taking the stairs instead of the elevator, walking or cycling instead of driving short distances, or doing household chores.

Remember, the goal is to move your body in a way that feels good and is sustainable for the long haul.

B. Strategies for Overcoming Challenges and Setbacks:

Weight loss journeys are rarely smooth sailing. There will be challenges and setbacks along the way, but it's essential not to let them derail your progress. Here are some strategies for overcoming common obstacles:

1. Set realistic goals: Unrealistic expectations can lead to frustration and disappointment. Set small, achievable goals and celebrate your progress along the way.

2. Identify triggers: Pay attention to what triggers unhealthy eating habits or derails your exercise routine. Once you identify these triggers, develop strategies to cope with them effectively.

3. Practice self-compassion: Be kind to yourself when facing setbacks. Instead of dwelling on mistakes, focus on what you can learn from them and move forward with renewed determination.

4. Seek support: Surround yourself with a supportive network of friends, family, or a professional coach who can offer encouragement and accountability.

Remember, setbacks are a natural part of the journey. What's important is how you respond to them and keep moving forward.

C. Importance of Self-Care and Mental Well-Being:

Weight loss isn't just about the number on the scale; it's about nourishing your body and mind. Prioritizing self-care and mental well-being is crucial for long-term success. Here's how you can take care of yourself:

1. Practice mindfulness: Pay attention to your body's hunger and fullness cues, and eat mindfully without distractions. Mindfulness techniques such as meditation and deep breathing can also help reduce stress and emotional eating.

2. Get enough sleep: Lack of sleep can disrupt hunger hormones and increase cravings for unhealthy foods. Aim for seven to eight hours of quality sleep each night to support your weight loss efforts.

3. Manage stress: Chronic stress can sabotage your weight loss goals by triggering emotional eating and disrupting sleep patterns. Find healthy ways to manage stress, such as exercise, meditation, or spending time in nature.

4. Take time for yourself: Make self-care a priority by engaging in activities that nourish your soul, whether it's reading a book, taking a bath, or spending time with loved ones.

Remember, sustainable weight loss is not just about changing your body; it's about transforming your lifestyle in a way that enhances your overall well-being. By incorporating physical activity, overcoming challenges with resilience, and prioritizing self-care and mental well-being, you can achieve lasting success on your weight loss journey.

In conclusion, "NOOM Diet Recipes" serves as a comprehensive guide to adopting a healthier lifestyle through mindful nutrition. Throughout this book, we've explored the diverse array of benefits that come with incorporating NOOM diet recipes into our daily lives. From weight management to improved energy levels, from enhanced mood to better overall health, the advantages are numerous and impactful.

Recapitulating the Benefits:

A. By embracing NOOM diet recipes, we've learned to make smarter food choices that nourish our bodies and minds. These recipes emphasize nutrient-dense ingredients, balanced proportions, and mindful eating practices, all of which contribute to improved health outcomes.

B. Moreover, this journey isn't merely about following a set of recipes; it's about fostering a culture of exploration and experimentation with healthy eating. As we've discovered, there's a wealth of flavors, textures, and cuisines waiting to be explored within the framework of the NOOM diet. Through continued exploration, we can expand our culinary horizons and discover new favorite dishes that support our well-being.

Encouragement for Continued Exploration:

C. As we conclude this journey, I encourage you to continue your exploration of healthy eating. Whether it's trying out new ingredients, experimenting with different cooking methods, or incorporating more plant-based meals into your diet, every step forward is a step toward better health. Remember that progress is a journey, not a destination, and each choice you make contributes to your overall well-being.

In the pursuit of a healthier lifestyle, it's essential to recognize the importance of balance. While nutrition is a fundamental aspect of our well-being, it's equally vital to nourish our minds and spirits. Cultivating a holistic approach to health involves not only what we eat but also how we move, how we rest, and how we care for ourselves emotionally and spiritually.

By embracing the principles of mindful nutrition outlined in this book, we take a significant step toward achieving that balance. We nourish our bodies with wholesome foods, honor our hunger and fullness cues, and cultivate a positive relationship with food. In doing so, we not only improve our physical health but also enhance our overall quality of life.

In closing, I hope that "NOOM Diet Recipes" has provided you with both inspiration and practical tools to embark on your journey toward better health. Remember that every small change you make has the potential to create a ripple effect of positive transformation in your life. Here's to your health, happiness, and continued exploration of the wonderful world of nutritious eating. Cheers to a vibrant, fulfilling life fueled by the power of NOOM diet recipes!

THE END

www.ingramcontent.com/pod-product-compliance
Lightning Source LLC
Chambersburg PA
CBHW061307250726
48653CB00002B/821